Acceptance and Commitment Therapy in 7 weeks .

A Complete Guide To Mindfulness Change And Recover From Anxiety, Depression, Panick Attacks, And Ange

Rose Mathis

the actions taken outside of their direct purview. Regardless, there are zero scenarios where the original author or the Publisher can be deemed liable in any fashion for any damages or hardships that may result from any of the information discussed herein.

Additionally, the information in the following pages is intended only for informational purposes and should thus be thought of as universal. As befitting its nature, it is presented without assurance regarding its prolonged validity or interim quality. Trademarks that are mentioned are done without written consent and can in no way be considered an endorsement from the trademark holder.

CHAPTER ONE

INTRODUCTION TO ACCEPTANCE AND COMMITMENT THERAPY (ACT).

INTRODUCTION

For quite a long time, specialists in the field of psychology have attempted to create science-based, time-restricted mediations for individuals who wish to beat emotional wellness conditions. Thus, numerous individuals have had huge achievement intending to and dealing with a scope of concerns and experience more prominent prosperity, therefore. In any case, long term recuperation and anticipation of relapse stay critical as territories of potential trouble for those looking for treatment for emotional wellness conditions. As of late, new sorts of nursing, including ACT, have been created with expectations of expanding long term achievement in the treatment of psychological well-being conditions.

The ACT is based on the social edge hypothesis (also known as relational frame theory (RFT)), a school of research concentrating on human language and insight. RFT proposes the sane aptitudes utilized by the human brain to tackle issues might be ineffectual in helping individuals defeat mental pains. Based on this recommendation, ACT treatment was created to instruct individuals that albeit mental agony is ordinary, and we can learn approaches to live more advantageous and healthier, by changing how we consider or think about pains.

Starting in the late 1990s, many treatment manuals have been created to plot approaches to utilize ACT to treat different psychological wellness conditions. Treatment using these manuals has been looked into experimentally. It has created support for the utilization of ACT in the treatment of substance abuse, psychosis, anxiety, depression, chronic pain, and eating disorders.

We formally state ACT as "act" and not as the initials A-C-T. There's a valid justification for this. At its centre, the ACT is a conduct treatment: it's tied in with making a move. In any case, it's not about simply any old action. In the first place, it's about qualities guided action. There's a major existential part to this model: What would you like to stand for in life? The main thing, somewhere down in your heart? What would you like to be associated with at your burial service? ACT gets you in contact with the main thing in the 10,000-foot view: your heart's most profound wants for whom you need to be and what you need to do during your short timeframe on this planet. You, at that point, utilize these fundamental beliefs to direct, persuade, and rouse conduct change. Second, it's about "careful" action: action that you take deliberately, with full mindfulness—open to your experience and completely occupied with whatever you're doing.

ACT gets its name from one of its centre messages: acknowledge what is out of your control, and focus on making a move that improves your life. The point of ACT is to assist us with creating a rich, full, and significant life while tolerating the pain that life unavoidably brings.

ACT does this by showing us mental abilities to handle painful considerations and emotions successfully so that they have considerably less impact and impact.

These are known as care aptitudes, and helping us to explain what's genuinely essential and significant to us—that is, explain our qualities—and utilize that information to direct, rouse, and inspire us to set objectives and make a move that advances or enrich our lives.

Not many individuals come to ACT and make a plunge headfirst. You, like most others, may start by plunging a toe in the water. Next, you put an entire foot in, at that point a knee, a whole leg. Presently you end up right now, with one leg in the water and one leg out. And by and large, you remain there for a long time, half, down the middle out, not exactly sure if ACT is for you. At long last, at some point, you dive in. And when you do as such, you find the water is warm, inviting, and animating; you feel free, light, and ingenious; and you need to invest significantly more energy in it. When this occurs, there's commonly no returning to your old method for working. (So if this hasn't just transpired, I trust it will before the finish of this book.) One explanation behind this underlying uncertainty about ACT is that it challenges the tried and true way of thinking and overturns the standard procedures of most Western psychology. For instance, most models of treatment are incredibly centred on indication (symptoms) decrease. They will suppose that customers need to reduce their side effects before they can have a superior existence.ACT takes a fundamentally extraordinary position. ACT expects that:

- Personal satisfaction is needy upon careful, values-guided action, and
- This is conceivable paying little heed to what number of signs you have—given that you react to your indications with care.

To put it another way, careful, values-consistent living is the ideal result in ACT, not side effect decrease. So even though ACT ordinarily diminishes signs, this is never the objective. (Incidentally, as "values-compatible living" is somewhat of a significant piece, for the majority of the book, I'll shorten it to "esteemed living." Sorry, I know it's not incredible English.) Thus in ACT, when we show a customer care abilities, the point isn't to diminish his signs; however, to permanently change his relationship with his side effects, so they never again keep him away from esteemed living. The fact that his side effects lessen is viewed as a "reward" as opposed to the central matter of treatment.

We don't state to our customers, "We're not going to attempt to decrease your side effects!" Why not? Since:

- This would set up a wide range of pointless helpful boundaries, and
- We realize that the side effect decrease is amazingly likely. (Despite the fact that we never focus on it, in pretty much every preliminary, what's It All About? and concentrate at any point done on the ACT, there is a noteworthy indication decrease—albeit in some cases it happens more gradually than in different models.)

So this means, on the off chance that you come to ACT from models that are extremely centred around attempting to diminish side effects, it's genuinely an enormous change in perspective. Fortunately, the vast majority—advisors and customers the same—think that it is a freeing one.

Notwithstanding, because ACT is so unique to other mental methodologies, numerous practitioners at first feel ungainly, on edge, helpless, confounded, or deficient. The uplifting news is ACT gives you the way to handle those flawlessly normal sentiments successfully. And the more you practice ACT on yourself to improve and upgrade your own life and to determine your painful issues, the more successful you'll be in applying it with your customers. Thus, enough of the prelude: we should begin!

ACCEPTANCE AND COMMITMENT THERAPY (ACT)

The ACT is one of the 'third wave' psychological and conduct treatments. It consolidates acknowledgement and care procedures close by change systems, in acknowledgement that change isn't always conceivable or attractive.

The ACT is hypothetically gotten from relational frame theory (RFT), which is a systematic conduct record of the functional properties of human language.

The ACT approach suggests that pains and brokenness emerge from endeavours to control or dispose of awkward encounters.

Endeavours to control or maintain a strategic distance from them can prompt the confusing impact of more prominent pains and an impression of loss of control of the concentration for elimination.

The point of ACT is to increment mental adaptability, which is characterized as "contacting the present minute completely as a cognizant individual, and dependent on what the circumstance bears, changing or enduring in conduct in the administration of chosen esteems."

PROCESSES OFACCEPTANCE AND COMMITMENT THERAPY (ACT)

The general objective of ACT is to increment psychological flexibility – the capacity to contact the present minute all the more completely as a cognizant person and to change or persevere in conduct while doing so serves esteemed closures. Psychological flexibility is set up through six centre ACT forms. Every one of these zones is conceptualized as a positive psychological attitude, not simply a strategy for staying away from psychopathology.

Acceptance

Acceptanceis educated as an option in contrast to experiential evasion. Acceptance includes the active and mindful grasp of those private occasions occasioned by one's history without superfluous endeavours to change their recurrence or structure, particularly while doing so would cause psychological damage. For instance, tension patients are educated to feel nervousness, as an inclination, completely and without protection; pains patients are given strategies that urge them to relinquish a battle with pains, etc. Acceptance (and defusion) in the ACT isn't an end in itself. Or maybe acceptance is encouraged as a strategy for expanding esteems based action.

Cognitive Defusion

Cognitive defusionstrategies endeavour to change the unfortunate elements of contemplations and other private occasions, as opposed to attempting to adjust their structure, recurrence, or situational affectability. Said another way, ACT endeavours to change how one interacts with or identifies with contemplations by making settings in which their unhelpful capacities are lessened. There are scores of such strategies that have been produced for a wide assortment of clinical introductions. For instance, a negative idea could be observed impartially, rehashed for all to hear until its sound remains, or treated as a remotely watched occasion by giving it a shape, size, shading, speed, or structure. An individual could thank their brain for such an intriguing idea, name the way toward intuition ("I have the idea that I am nothing worth mentioning"), or look at the recorded contemplations, sentiments, and recollections that happen while they experience that idea. Such strategies endeavour to lessen the precise nature of the idea, debilitating the inclination to regard the idea as what it alludes to ("I am nothing worth mentioning") instead of what it is legitimately experienced to be (e.g., the idea "I am a whole lot of nothing"). The consequence of defusion is generally decreased inauthenticity of, or connection to, private occasions as opposed to a quick change in their recurrence.

Being Present

It advances continuous non-critical contact with psychological and natural occasions as they happen. The objective is to have customers experience the world all the more legitimately, so their conduct is progressively adaptable, and in this way, their actions increasingly predictable with the qualities that they hold. This is cultivated by permitting usefulness to apply more authority over conduct; and by utilizing language more as a device to note and depict occasions, not just to foresee and pass judgment on them. A feeling of self-called "self as a procedure" is actively energized: the defused, non-critical progressing depiction of considerations, sentiments, and other private occasions.

Self Context

This is a consequence of relational frames, for example, I versus You, Now versus Then, and Here versus There, human language prompts a feeling of self as a locus or point of view, and gives an extraordinary, profound side to ordinary verbal people. This thought was one of the seeds from which both the ACT and RFT developed, and there is currently developing proof of its significance to language capacities, for example, sympathy, theory of the brain, feeling of self, and such. In a word the thought is that "I" develops over huge arrangements of models of viewpoint taking relations, however since this feeling of self is a context for verbal knowing, not the substance of that knowing, it's cutoff points can't be deliberately known. Self as the context is significant to some degree because, from this point of view, one can understand one's progression of encounters without connection to them or an interest in which specific encounters happen: in this manner,defusion and acceptance are cultivated. Self as context is encouraged in the ACT by care activities, analogies, and experiential procedures.

Qualities Or Values

Qualities or values are selected characteristics of purposive action that can never be seen as an object; however,it can be launched minute by minute. ACT utilizes an assortment of activities to enable a customer to pick life bearings in different spaces (for example family, vocation, otherworldliness) while undermining verbal procedures that may prompt decisions dependent on evasion, social consistency, or combination (for example "I should value X" or "A great individual would value Y" or "My mom needs me to value Z"). In ACT, acceptance, defusion, being available, etc. are not finishes in themselves; instead, they make way for an increasingly fundamental, values, reliable life.

Committed Action

Finally, ACT energizes the improvement of more prominent and more significant examples of viable action connected to picked esteems. Right now, looks especially like conventional conduct treatment, and practically any typically cognizant conduct change strategy can be fitted into an ACT convention, including introduction, abilities obtaining, moulding strategies, objective setting, and so forth. In contrast to values, which are continually launched, however, never accomplished as an article, solid objectives that value predicted can be achieved, and ACT conventions quite often include treatment work and schoolwork connected to short, medium, and long term conduct change objectives. Conduct change endeavours thus lead to contact with psychological obstructions that are tended to through other ACT forms (acceptance, defusion, etc.).

HOW ACT WORKS

People are the main creature ready to make connections(relationships) among words and thoughts. For instance, we can relate apples and oranges to the general idea of natural products. While this is unfathomably valuable for preparing our general surroundings, it can make issues when we partner harmless thoughts in a negative example. After some time, individuals can start to relate ideas like disappointment or uselessness to themselves, setting them up for progressively negative results later on.

ACT works by instructing patients to recognize and proceed onward from these points of view, instead of permitting them to get imbued. While pessimistic considerations can be reasonable and proper reactions to specific circumstances, they don't characterize who an individual is as an individual, and ought not to keep that individual from proceeding onward with their life.

At the point when you see a specialist for the ACT, you'll start by figuring out how to tune in to how you converse with yourself, called self-talk. The principle centre will be your self-talk encompassing awful mishaps and other harmful parts of your life, as undesirable connections, physical issues, and then some. Your specialist will, at that point, assist you with deciding if these perspectives are things that you can change, such as leaving acomplicated relationship, or that you should acknowledge how they are, similar to a physical incapacity. If you can change the circumstance, your specialist will assist you with creating techniques for making the essential changes throughout your life as per your objectives and qualities. On the off chance that the issue is something that you can't transform, you can start to learn social techniques to work around your difficulties, so they don't have as quite a bit of a negative impact on your life.

When you have understood the present significant issues throughout your life, you and your specialist can start to assess any examples that have developed from quite a while ago. Along these lines, you can abstain from rehashing any negative patterns later on. Instead of battling with your feelings, you can figure out how to recognize them for what they are and figure out how to function with or around them to accomplish the satisfying life you need.

BENEFIT OF ACT

The critical advantage of ACT is that it can assist patients with doing combating mental clutters like tension and melancholy without utilizing medicine. It trains patients to change how they identify with their negative musings and feelings, so these considerations don't dominate. While patients will be unable to dispose of every single pharmaceutical drug immediately, they might have the option to decrease their dose after some time, at last going off the prescription. With the narcotic emergency being such an intriguing issue in the clinical and psychological fields, it is promising to have compelling treatment choices that don't require drugs.

At its most essential level, ACT urges patients to acknowledge those things that are out of their control and focus on different contemplations and actions intended to improve their lives. Instead of feeling remorseful about having negative considerations or sentiments, patients discover that negative feelings are superbly common. At the point when they can acknowledge the negative pieces of their awareness, patients are all the more allowed to begin moving endlessly from them and towards a progressively positive course. The objective of ACT is to increment psychological flexibility. Practitioners assist patients with getting increasingly mindful of the manners in which they think and feel through care activities and techniques. They additionally centre around making enduring conduct changes by focusing on new actions and considered designs. Patients figure out how to acknowledge their contemplations as they are and to assess those musings to decide if they are serving the patient's life objectives. On the off chance that the contemplations are not helping them, patients can work to ingrain new, progressively positive considerations and actions.

Acceptance and Commitment Therapy (ACT) is a special type of therapy that urges patients to grasp their negative musings and sentiments as opposed to attempting to keep away from or dispense with them. Prepared specialists utilize this strategy to treat a broad scope of conditions, and it has demonstrated to be surprisingly powerful for some individuals.

MINDFULNESS AND ACT

Mindfulness is portrayed as keeping in touch with the present minute as opposed to floating off into a programmed pilot. Mindfulness permits a person to interface with the watching self, the part they know about, however, separate from the reasoning self. Mindfulness methods frequently assist individuals with expanding attention to every one of the five faculties just as of their contemplations and feelings.

Mindfulness likewise builds a person's capacity to withdraw from contemplations. Moves identified with painful emotions, desires, or circumstances are frequently first decreased and afterward, in the long run, acknowledged. Acceptance is the capacity to permit interior and outer experience to happen as opposed to battling or maintaining a strategic distance from the experience. On the off chance that somebody believes, "I'm a horrible individual," that individual may be asked instead to say, "I have the idea that I'm an awful individual." This adequately isolates the individual from the perception, subsequently stripping it of its negative charge.

At the point when individuals experience excruciating feelings, for example, tension, they may be told to open up, breathe into, or make space for the physical sentiment of uneasiness and permit it to stay there; similarly, all things considered, without fueling or limiting it.

THEORY OF ACT

ACT theory doesn't characterize awkward enthusiastic encounters as indications or issues. It instead attempts to address the propensity of some to see people who look for therapy as harmed or imperfect and means to assist individuals with understanding the totality and essentialness of life. This totality incorporates a wide range of human experience, including the agony unavoidably going with specific circumstances.

Acceptance of astonishingly, without assessing or endeavouring to transform them, is expertise created through mindfulness practices all through the meeting. ACT doesn't attempt to legitimately change or stop undesirable musings or sentiments (as cognitive conduct therapy does) yet instead urges individuals to build up another and loving relationship with those encounters. This move can liberate individuals from troubles endeavouring to control their encounters and assist them with getting increasingly open to actions reliable with their qualities, values explanation, and the meaning of qualities based objectives additionally being key parts of ACT.

OBJECTIVE OF ACT

ACT aims to make a rich and significant life while tolerating the pains that unavoidably goes with it. "ACT" is a decent truncation, since this therapy is tied in with making compelling move guided by our most profound qualities and in which we are completely present and locked in. It is just through careful action that we can make a valuable life. As we endeavour to make such a real existence, we will experience a wide range of boundaries, as horrendous and undesirable "private encounters" (thoughts, images, feelings, sensations, urges, and memories). ACT arrives at mindfulness aptitudes as a successful method to deal with these private encounters.

CHAPTER TWO

DEPRESSION

Depression is a typical sickness around the world, with over 264 million individuals influenced. Depression is unique concerningnormal mindset variances and fleeting passionate reactions to challenges in regular day to day existence. Particularly when dependable and with moderate or extreme force, depression may turn into a good wellbeing condition. It can make the influenced individual endure incredibly and work ineffectively, grinding away, at school, and in the family. From a pessimistic standpoint, depression can prompt suicide. Near 800 000 individuals kick the bucket because of suicide consistently. Suicide is the following driving reason for death in 15-29-year-olds. Even though there are known, successful medicines for mental disarranges, somewhere in the range of 76% and 85% of individuals in low-and centre pay nations to get no treatment for their confusion. Hindrances to viable consideration incorporate an absence of assets, absence of prepared medicinal services suppliers, and social disgrace related to mental issues. Another obstruction to viable consideration is off base evaluation. In nations of all salary levels, individuals who are discouraged are regularly not effectively analyzed, and other people who don't have the turmoil are again and again misdiagnosed and endorsed antidepressants. The weight of depression and other psychological wellness conditions is on the ascent, all-inclusive.

CAUSES OF DEPRESSION

Various components may expand the opportunity of grief, including the accompanying:

Abuse.

Past physical, sexual, or psychological mistreatment can expand the helplessness to clinical sorrow sometime down the road.

Certain drugs.

A few medications, for example, isotretinoin (used to treat skin inflammation), the antiviral medication interferon-alpha, and corticosteroids, can expand your danger of misery.

Conflict.

Despondency in somebody who has the organic helplessness to create sorrow may result from individual clashes or questions with relatives or companions.

Death or a misfortune.

Trouble or melancholy from the passing or loss of a friend or family member, however characteristic may expand the danger of misery.

Genetics.

A family ancestry of sorrow may be hazardous. It's idea that a downturn is a perplexing characteristic, implying that there is likely a wide range of qualities that each apply little impacts instead of a solitary quality that adds to sickness hazard. The hereditary conditions of misery, likemost mental issues, are not as necessary or direct as in absolutely genetic ailments, for example, Huntington's chorea or cystic fibrosis.

Major occasions.

Indeed, even great occasions, for example, beginning a new position, graduating, or getting hitched can prompt sadness. So can moving, losing a vocation or salary, getting separated, or resigning. Be that as it may, the disorder of clinical sorrow is never only an "ordinary" reaction to distressing life occasions.

Other individual issues.

Issues, for example, social disconnection because of other psychological maladjustments or being thrown out of a family or social gathering, can add to the danger of creating clinical sadness.

Serious diseases.

Now and then,sadness exists together with a significant ailment or might be activated by another medical condition.

Substance misuse.

Almost 30% of individuals with substance misuse issues likewise have significant or clinical despondency. Regardless of whether medications or liquor incidentally cause you to feel better, they, at last, will disturb wretchedness.

Family history.

You're at a higher hazard for creating misery on the off chance that you have a family ancestry of gloom or another disposition issue.

Early youth trauma.

A few occasions influence how your body responds to fear and upsetting circumstances.

Brain structure.

There's a more severe hazard for gloom if the frontal projection of your brain is less dynamic. Be that as it may, researchers don't have the foggiest idea whether this occurs previously or after the beginning of burdensome signs.

Medical conditions.

Certain conditions may put you at higher hazard, for example, interminable disease, a sleeping disorder, constantpains, or attention-deficit hyperactivity disorder (ADHD).

TIERS OF DEPRESSION

Major Depression (Clinical Depression)

Major burdensome issue, otherwise called unipolar or clinical depression, is described by a tenacious sentiment of trouble or an absence of enthusiasm for outside upgrades. You may have this kind of depression if you have at least five of the accompanying side effects on most days for about fourteen days or longer. At any rate, one of the side effects must be in a discouraged state of mind or loss of enthusiasm for exercises.

- Loss of interest or in your activities
- Feelings of worthlessness or guilt
- Negative thinking with an inability to see positive solutions
- Feeling restless or agitated
- Inability to focus
- Lashing out at loved ones
- Irritability
- Withdrawing from loved ones
- Increase in sleeping

- Exhaustion and lethargy
- Morbid, suicidal thoughts
- Weight loss or gain

What is a major depressive scene or episode?

A major depressive scene is a time of about fourteen days or longer in which an individual encounters the side effects of major depression, for example, sadness, loss of delight, weakness, and self-destructive contemplations. Specifically, the individual must experience a low mind-set and additionally lost enthusiasm for exercises.

Is a major depressive issue curable?

The major depressive issue is a condition that can make rhythmic movement over an individual's lifetime. The major depressive issue is along these lines not considered "curable," yet with the correct treatment, the side effects of depression can be overseen and mitigated after some time.

What is the best treatment for the major depressive issue?

An assortment of treatment choices is accessible for a major depressive issue, including psychotherapy, energizer meds, psychological conduct treatment, electroconvulsive treatment (ECT), and regular medicines. The treatment plan will vary for every individual relying upon singular needs; however, the "best" treatment for major depressive issue is regularly thought to be a blend of medicine and therapy.

Dysthymia (Persistent Depressive Disorder)

Dysthymia, otherwise called a persistent depressive disorder, is a long term type of depression that goes on for a considerable length of time and can meddle with everyday life, work, and connections. Individuals with dysthymia frequently think that its hard to be cheerful even on commonly blissful events. They might be seen as bleak, negative, or a whiner when, as a general rule, they are managing an incessant psychological mal-adjustment. Side effects of dysthymia can go back and forth after some time, and the force of the side effects can change, yet side effects, for the most part, don't vanish for over two months one after another.

How is dysthymia unique related to major depression?

The depressed state of mind experienced with dysthymia isn't as dangerous as major depressive disorder, yet brings out sentiments of trouble, misery, and loss of delight. While the side effects of depression must be available for at any rate two weeks to be determined to have major depressive disorder, a determination of dysthymia requires having encountered a mix of depressive side effects for a long time or more.

What is implied by "advanced" depression?

The term advanced depression is frequently used to refers to dysthymia, or persistent depressive disorder, as because of the interminable idea of this kind of depression, numerous people living with the disorder keep on making an insincere effort of life in an automated manner, apparently fine to everyone around them.

What is two fold depression?

Twofold depression is a complexity of dysthymia. After some time, the more significant part of individuals with dysthymia experience exacerbating side effects that lead to the beginning of a full disorder of major depression over their dysthymic disorder, bringing about what is known as twofold depression.

Manic Depression (Bipolar Disorder)

Bipolar disorder, at times alluded to as manic depression, is a psychological well-being condition that causes outrageous variances in mind-set and changes in vitality, thinking, conduct, and rest. With manic depression, you don't simply feel "sad;"

your depressive state may prompt self-destructive considerations that change over to sentiments of happiness and perpetual vitality. These extraordinary emotional episodes can happen all the more much of the time, for example, consistently or show up sporadically–perhaps just two times every year. Mind-set stabilizers, for example, lithium, can be utilized to control the emotional episodes that accompany the bipolar disorder, yet people are likewise recommended a wide range of meds, including antidepressants and atypical antipsychotics.

Is bipolar disorder hereditary?

While researchers have not pinpointed one single main driver, it shows up hereditary qualities are probably going to represent around 60-80% of the hazard for creating bipolar disorder, demonstrating the key role heredity plays right now. Your danger of creating bipolar disorder is additionally expanded essentially on the off chance that you have a first-degree relative experiencing the disorder.

Can bipolar disorder be cured?

Presently, there is no remedy for bipolar disorder, yet it very well may be overseen effectively with a treatment plan, including a mix of medicine and psychotherapy.

What's the distinction between bipolar 1 and bipolar 2 disorder?

While a wide range of bipolar disorder includes extraordinary highs and lows, the fundamental distinction between bipolar 1 and bipolar 2 is the seriousness of the manic indications. With bipolar 1,the insanity, or raised temperament, usually is more severe than with bipolar 2. With bipolar 2, the individual encounters hypomania, a less severe type of lunacy that brings about practices that are atypical for the individual yet not irregular to society on the loose.

Postpartum Depression (Peripartum Depression)

Tragic sentiments and crying sessions that follow labour are known as "postnatal anxiety." postnatal depression is normal and will, in general,decrease inside up to 14 days. This kind of misery is regularly credited to the emotional, hormonal changes that follow labour. Around one out of seven ladies will encounter something more extraordinary than the run of the postnatal mill anxiety. In any case, ladies that conceive an offspring and battle with bitterness, tension, or stress for half a month or more may have postpartum depression (PPD). Signs and side effects of PPD include:

- Feeling down or discouraged for a large portion of the day for half a month or more
- Feeling far off and pulled back from loved ones

- A loss of enthusiasm for exercises (including sex)
- Changes in eating and dozing propensities
- Feeling tired a large portion of the day
- Feeling furious or fractious
- Having sentiments of tension, stress, alarm assaults or dashing musings

Can postpartum depression start a very long time after conceiving an offspring?

Postpartum depression doesn't start quickly following the introduction of an infant. Postpartum depression signs may begin in the initial barely any weeks following labour; however, in some cases, side effects of PPD don't start until months after birth and can develop whenever during the child's first year.

Why does postpartum depression happen?

While the specific reason for postpartum depression is obscure, it is believed to be a consequence of an assortment of components including the physical changes coming about because of pregnancy; tension about parenthood; hormonal changes; past psychological well-being issues; absence of help; a confused pregnancy or conveyance, and additionally changes to the rest cycle.

Can postpartum depression go back and forth?

"Ladies who have experienced postpartum depression (PPD) are consistently in danger for future temperament scenes from that point the primary experience of depression, possibly since the "switch" for having those scenes is currently flipped after the PPD, and since the pressure of parenthood doesn't leave and can even exacerbate contingent upon mental stressors that are continuous," says Jean Kim, M.D. "On the off chance that the lady is taking drug for the depressive signs it might lose adequacy for reasons unknown at a while out, so it wouldn't be incomprehensible for a backslide to happen a while after the underlying PPD scene."

Seasonal Affective Disorder (SAD)

Seasonal affective disorder (SAD) is a kind of depression identified with the difference in season. Individuals who experience the ill effects of SAD notification signs starting and completion at about similar occasions every year. For some, symptoms begin in the fall and proceed into the winter months; however, it is workable for SAD to happen in the spring or summer. In either case, indications of depression, for example, sadness, exhaustion, and loss of intrigue or joy in exercises, begin mellow and progress to be increasingly dangerous as the weeks go on. The individuals who experience SAD in the winter have likewise noticed the accompanying one of a kind side effects:

- Heaviness in arms and legs
- Frequent sleeping late
- Cravings for starches/weight gain
- Relationship issues

How is seasonal affective disorder (SAD) treated?

Treatment plans for seasonal affective disorder (SAD) may incorporate medicine, psychotherapy, light treatment, or a mix of these alternatives to deal with the depression signs. Talk treatment can be a priceless choice for those with SAD. A psychotherapist can assist you with recognizing designs in contrary reasoning and conduct that sway depression, learn positive methods for adapting to signs, and establishment unwinding strategies that can help you with reestablishing lost vitality.

Can seasonal affective disorder occur in the late spring?

Seasonal affective disorder (SAD) in the late spring months is more typical than you may suspect. Around 10% of people with

SAD start seeing the indications of depression in the late spring months.

Why does seasonal affective disorder happen?

The specific reason for seasonal affective disorder (SAD) is as yet misty; however, specialists have made an assortment of theories identified with the reason for the disorder and why some experience more extreme side effects than others. It has been recommended that the impacts of light, a disturbed body clock, low serotonin levels, high melatonin levels, awful life occasions, and even physical ailment are associated with the beginning of SAD.

Psychotic Depression

As indicated by the National Alliance on Mental Illness, around 20 percent of individuals with depression have scenes so severe that they create psychotic side effects. A finding of major depressive disorder with psychotic highlights might be given to people experiencing a blend of the signs of depression and psychosis: a psychological state portrayed by scattered reasoning or conduct; deceptions, known as daydreams, or bogus sights or sounds, known as mind flights.

What are the early indications of psychosis?

Early psychosis alludes to the period when an individual first begins to seem like they are losing contact with the real world.

The initial indications of psychosis incorporate doubt of others, pulling back socially, serious and unseemly feelings, inconvenience thinking plainly, a decrease in close to home cleanliness and a drop in execution busy working or school.

How is psychotic depression analyzed?

To be determined to have major depressive disorder with psychotic highlights, the individual must have a depressive scene that endures two weeks or more and be encountering dreams and visualizations. There are two distinct kinds of major depressive disorder with psychotic highlights, the two of which noticeably include dreams and mental trips. Individual experience major depressive disorder with state of mind compatible psychotic highlights (the substance of the fantasies and daydreams is predictable with depressive subjects) or with mind-set incongruent psychotic highlights (the content of the pipedreams and dreams doesn't include depressive topics).

Can psychotic depression transform into schizophrenia?

Depression is a mind-set disorder and schizophrenia is a psychotic ailment; while both psychotic depression and schizophrenia share psychosis as a side effect, there is no motivation to believe that psychotic depression would transform into schizophrenia. Alternately, people with schizophrenia can become discouraged when they understand the disgrace encompassing their disease, poor forecast, and loss of capacity.

Premenstrual Dysphoric Disorder (PMDD)

Premenstrual dysphoric disorder, or PMDD, is a cyclic, hormone-based disposition disorder, regularly thought to be an extreme and debilitating type of premenstrual syndrome (PMS). While up to 85% of ladies experience PMS, just around 5% of ladies are determined to have PMDD, as indicated by an examination in the American Journal of Psychiatry. While the centre indications of PMDD identify with discouraged temperament and nervousness, conduct and physical signs additionally happen. To get a determination of PMDD, a lady more likely than not experienced symptoms during the more significant part of the menstrual patterns of the previous year and these side effects probably adversely affected work or social working.

What is the distinction between PMDD and PMS?

Premenstrual dysphoric disorder (PMDD) is a more genuine condition than premenstrual syndrome (PMS). The indications present with PMS don't come by, and large meddle with ordinary capacity and are less extreme in their force. While it is typical for ladies to encounter change in temperament in the days paving the way to period, the mental side effects of severe depression, tension, and self-destructive musings don't happen with PMS.

What is the best medicine for PMDD?

For the side effects of PMDD identified with mind-set and uneasiness, a gathering of antidepressants named specific serotonin reuptake inhibitors (SSRIs) can be endorsed; sertraline, fluoxetine, and paroxetine hydrochloride have all been affirmed by the FDA as drugs which might be recommended to ease pains.

How long do PMDD side effects last?

The indications of premenstrual dysphoric disorder (PMDD) commonly reoccur every month before and during the feminine cycle. Side effects usually start 7-10 days before the female cycle and decrease in power inside a couple of days of the period beginning. Side effects vanish totally until the following premenstrual stage.

Atypical Depression

Regardless of its name, atypical depression may in certainty be one of the most noticeable sorts of depression. Atypical depression is not quite the same as the steady bitterness or sadness that describes major depression. It is viewed as a "specifier" or subtype of major depression that depicts an example of depression side effects, including sleeping in, gorging, peevishness, weight in the arms and legs, affectability to dismissal, and relationship issues. One of the first signs of atypical depression is the capacity for the state of mind of the discouraged individual to improve following a favourable occasion.

How genuine is atypical depression?

Similarly, likewise, with a depression, atypical depression is a positive psychological well-being condition and is related to an expanded danger of suicide and tension disorders. Atypical depression regularly begins in the adolescent years, sooner than different kinds of depression, and can have an all the more long term (constant) course.

How do you treat atypical depression?

Atypical depression reacts well to treatment contained the two drugs and psychotherapy. Monoamine oxidase inhibitors (MAOIs) and different antidepressants, for example, SSRIs and tricyclic antidepressants are the most widely recognized meds recommended to treat atypical depression.

Can atypical depression be cured?

There is nobody size-fits-all treatment to "fix" atypical depression; however, it very well may be effectively made do with a mix of medicine and psychotherapy. Abatement is the objective for atypical depression; however, recollect that depression has a high danger of reoccurrence, so it is essential to be aware of any reappearing side effects.

Situational Depression (Reactive Depression/Adjustment Disorder)

Situational depression, also called responsive depression or modification disorder, is a present moment, stress-related sort of depression. It can create after an individual encounters an awful mishap or a progression of changes to their regular day to day existence. Instances of occasions or changes that may trigger situational depression incorporate, however, are not restricted to: separate, retirement, loss of a companion, disease, and relationship issues. Situational depression is in this manner a kind of modification disorder, as it originates from an individual's battle to grapple with the progressions that have happened. Many people who experience situational depression start to have signs inside around 90 days following the activating occasion.

How is situational depression not quite the same as clinical depression?

On the off chance that you have situational depression, you will encounter a large number of similar signs someone with major depressive disorder. The key contrast is situational depression is a momentary reaction activated by an occasion in somebody's life, and the symptoms will settle when the stressor never again exists, or the individual can adjust to the circumstance. Not at all like situational depression, major depressive disorder is viewed as a temperament disorder and usually includes awkward synthetic nature in the brain.

How is situational depression analyzed?

To be determined to have situational depression, an individual must encounter mental and conduct side effects inside three months of a recognizable stressor, that are past what might be viewed as a common reaction, and improve inside a half year after the aggressor is expelled.

Who is in danger of creating situational depression?

It is highly unlikely to foresee which individual out of a gathering of individuals encountering a similar stressor will create situational depression. However, it is accepted your social aptitudes before the occasion and how you manage pressure may assume a job.

Disruptive Mood Dysregulation Disorder (DMDD)

DMDD is a genuinely late determination, showing up without precedent for the Diagnostic and Statistical Manual of Mental Disorders (DSM-5) in 2013. The DSM-5 characterizes DMDD as a kind of burdensome disorder, as kids determined to have DMDD battle to manage their moods and feelings during a time fitting way. Accordingly, kids with DMDD display visit temper upheavals in light of dissatisfaction, either verbally or typically. In the middle of changes, they experience ceaseless, diligent fractiousness.

How is DMDD not the same as bipolar disorder?

While the vital element of DMDD is touchiness, the sign of the bipolar disorder is the nearness of hyper or hypomanic scenes. Even though DMDD and bipolar disorder can both reason touchiness, hyper scenes will, in general, happen sporadically, while in DMDD, the peevish mood is severe and ceaseless.

What is the treatment for DMDD?

A mix of psychotherapy and parent the board strategies is the initial move towards training kids adapting aptitudes for controlling their moods and feelings and showing guardians how to oversee upheavals. Nonetheless, a medicine may likewise be recommended if these strategies alone are not compelling.

Can youngsters develop out of DMDD?

Youngsters are probably not going to develop out of DMDD without figuring out how to control their moods and feelings adequately. On the off chance that you figure your kid may have DMDD, look for counsel from psychological wellness proficient for analysis and a viable treatment plan.

Living with depression can feel like a daunting task, yet it isn't something you need to confront alone. You can take our free, classified depression test, as a starter self-evaluation for the signs of depression.

It's critical to realize that physical sickness additionally expands the danger of creating severe burdensome ailment. Depression can be brought about by an entire assortment of ailments that impact the body's frameworks or from ceaseless ailments that cause continuous agony. It is exceptionally normal among the individuals who have diseases, for example, the accompanying:

- Cancer
- Coronary illness
- Diabetes
- Epilepsy

- Multiple sclerosis
- Stroke
- Alzheimer's sickness
- HIV/AIDS
- Systemic lupus erythematosus
- Rheumatoid joint pain

Additionally, depression can be instigated by specific substances and prescriptions, so be set up to have a transparent conversation with your psychological well-being proficient about your liquor consumption and any recommended or recreational medication use.

If you figure you might be experiencing any of these various kinds of depression, we encourage you to contact your PCP or a psychological wellness expert to get the determination, treatment, and bolster you need.

SIGNS AND SYMPTOMS OF DEPRESSION

Depression can be more than a consistent condition of bitterness or feeling "blue."

Significant depression can cause an assortment of indications. Some influence your mood, and others influence your body. Side effects may likewise be progressing, or travel every which way.

The side effects of depression can be experienced distinctively among men, ladies, and youngsters in an unexpected way.

Men may encounter side effects identified with their:

- Mood: for example, outrage, forcefulness, touchiness, uneasiness, anxiety
- Emotional prosperity: for instance, feeling vacant, miserable, and sad
- Behaviour: for example, loss of intrigue, never again discovering delight in most loved exercises, feeling tired effectively, considerations of suicide, drinking exorbitantly, utilizing drugs, participating in high-hazard exercises
- Sexual intrigue: for example, diminished sexual want, absence of sexual execution
- Cognitive capacities: for example, failure to focus, trouble finishing errands, postponed reactions during discussions
- Sleep designs: for example, a sleeping disorder, anxious rest, over the top tiredness, not staying asleep for the entire evening
- physical prosperity: for example, exhaustion, pains, migraine, stomach related issues.

Ladies may encounter side effects identified with their:

- mood: for example, crabbiness
- emotional prosperity: for instance, feeling tragic or vacant, on edge or sad
- Behaviour: for example, loss of enthusiasm for exercises, pulling back from social commitment, musings.
- cognitive capacities: for example, thinking or talking all the more gradually
- sleep designs: for example, trouble staying asleep for the entire evening, waking early, dozing excessively
- physical prosperity: for instance, diminished vitality, more prominent weariness, changes in hunger, weight changes, hurts, pains, migraines, expanded issues

Youngsters may encounter side effects identified with their:

- mood: for example, touchiness, outrage, mood swings, crying
- emotional prosperity: for example, sentiments of ineptitude (for instance "I can't do anything right") or hopelessness, crying, exceptional pity

- behaviour: for example, falling into difficulty at school or declining to go to class, evading companions or kin, musings of death or suicide
- cognitive capacities: for example, trouble concentrating, decrease in school execution, changes in grades

- sleep design: for example, difficultyin resting or dozing excessively
- physical prosperity: for example, loss of vitality, stomach related issues, changes in hunger, weight reduction or addition

CONDITIONS THAT GET WORSE DUE TO DEPRESSION

Here are conditions that can get worse due to depression: arthritis,asthma, cardiovascular illness, cancer,diabetes and obesity.

Arthritis

Arthritis is an aggravation of the joints. It can influence either one bone or various joints. There are more than 100 unique sorts of joint pain, with multiple causes and treatment techniques. Two of the most well-known kinds are osteoarthritis (OA) and rheumatoid joint inflammation(Also called Rheumatoid arthritis (RA).

The side effects of joint inflammation, as a rule, create after some time, yet they may likewise show up out of nowhere. Joint inflammation is most generally found in grown-ups beyond 65 years old, yet it can alsoaffect kids, adolescents, and adults. Joint pain is more typical in ladies than men and in individuals who are overweight.

Kinds of Arthritis

Osteoarthritis (OA) is a kind of common illness that outcomes from the breakdown of joint ligament and hidden bone. The most widely recognized indications are joint pains and firmness. Usually, the signs progress gradually over the years.

Rheumatoid joint pain is a long term, dynamic, and handicapping immune system infection. It causes irritation, growing, and pains in and around the joints and other body organs.

Rheumatoid joint inflammation, for the most part, influences the hands and feet first, yet it can happen in any joint. It, as a rule, includes similar joints on the two sides of the body.

Basic indications incorporate rigid joints, particularly after finding a workable pace morning or in the wake of plunking down for some time. A few people frequently experience weakness and a general sentiment of being unwell.

Causes joint inflammation

A ligament is a firm yet adaptable connective tissue in your joints. It secures the joints by engrossing the weight and stun made when you move and put pressure on them. A decrease in the standard measure of this ligament tissue causes a few types of joint inflammation.

Typical mileage causes OA, one of the most widely recognized types of joint pain. Contamination or injury to the joints can intensify this normal breakdown of ligament tissue. Your danger of creating OA might be higher on the off chance that you have a family ancestry of the ailment.

Another regular type of joint inflammation, RA, is an immune system disorder. It happens when your body's invulnerable framework assaults the tissues of the body. These assaults influence the synovium, a delicate tissue in your joints that delivers a liquid that feeds the ligament and greases up the bones.

RA is anillness of the synovium that will attack and decimate a joint. It can, in the end, lead to the pulverization of both bone and ligament inside the joint.

The specific reason for the resistant framework's assaults is obscure. Yet, researchers have found genetic markers that expansion your danger of creating RA fivefold.

The indications of joint pain

Joint pains, solidness, and growing are the most widely recognized side effects of joint inflammation. Your scope of movement may likewise diminish, and you may encounter redness of the skin around the joint. Numerous individuals with joint inflammation notice their side effects are more terrible toward the beginning of the day.

On account of RA, you may feel tired, or experience lost craving because of the irritation the resistant framework's movement causes. You may likewise get frail — which means your red platelet check diminishes — or have a slight fever. Severe RA can cause joint distortion whenever left untreated.

Asthma

Asthma is a long termillness of the lungs. You may hear your PCP consider it a persistent respiratory disease. It makes your aviation routes get excited and thin and makes breathing troublesome. Hacking, wheezing, the brevity of breath and chest snugness are exemplary asthma indications.

Components of asthma include:

- Genetics: If a parent has asthma, you're bound to create it.
- History of viral contaminations: Individuals with a background marked by viral diseases during youth are bound to build up the condition.
- Hygiene theory: This speculation suggests that children aren't presented to enough microbes in their initial months and years. Accordingly, their safe frameworks don't get sufficiently able to fend off asthma and different conditions.
- Early allergen presentation: Visit contact with potential allergens and aggravations may expand your hazard for creating asthma.

Side effects of asthma

- Illness: Respiratory sicknesses, for example, this season's cold virus and pneumonia can trigger asthma assaults.
- Exercise: Expanded development may make breathing progressively troublesome.
- Irritants noticeable all around: Individuals with asthma might be touchy to aggravations, for example, synthetic exhaust, solid scents, and smoke.

- Allergens: Animals dander, dust vermin, and dust are only a couple of instances of allergens that can trigger side effects.
- Extreme climate conditions: for example, high dampness or low temperatures may trigger asthma.
- Emotions: Yelling, chuckling, and crying may trigger an assault.

Cardiovascular illness

Cardiovascular illness which is otherwise called Heart ailment is the primary source of death on the planet at present, as indicated by the Centers for Disease Control and Prevention (CDCP)Trusted Source. In the World, 1 in each fourdeath in is the consequence of coronary illness. That is around 610,000 individuals who kick the bucket from the condition every year.

Coronary illness doesn't segregate. It's the main source of death for a few populaces, including Caucasians, Hispanics, and African-Americans. Practically 50% of Americans are in danger of coronary illness, and the numbers are rising.

While coronary illness can be destructive, it's likewise preventable in the vast majority. By embracing a reliable way of life propensities early, you can live longer with a more advantageous or healthy heart.

Symptoms of Cardiovascular illness

Cardiovascular illness indications might be diverse for people. For example, men are bound to have chest pains; ladies are bound to have different side effects alongside chest uneasiness, for instance, the brevity of breath, queasiness and extraordinary weariness.

Side effects can include:

- Chest pains, chest snugness, chest weight and chest inconvenience (angina)
- Shortness of breath
- Pain, shortcoming or chilliness in your legs or arms if the veins in those pieces of your body are limited
- Pain in the neck, jaw, throat, upper stomach area or back

Cancer

Cancer is a gathering of diseases including irregular cell development with the possibility to attack or spread to different pieces of the body. These stand out from amiable tumours, which don't spread.

Depression is very regular in individuals living with malignant growth. As indicated by the American Cancer Society, around 1 out of 4 individuals with the disease have clinical depression.

Clinical depression additionally referred to just as Major burdensome disorder (MDD), is a psychological disorder described by in any event two weeks of low mood that is available across most circumstances

A portion of the signs that malignant growth may cause include:

- Breast changes
- A lump or firm inclination in your breast or under your arm
- Nipple changes or release
- Skin that is bothersome, red, layered, dimpled, or puckered
- Bladder changes
- Trouble peeing
- Pain while peeing
- Blood in the pee
- Draining or wounding, for no known explanation

Entrails changes

- Blood in the stools
- Changes in entrail propensities
- Hack or roughness that doesn't leave
- Eating issues
- Pain in the wake of eating (acid reflux or heartburn that doesn't go)
- Trouble gulping
- Belly pains
- Nausea and spewing
- Appetite changes
- Exhaustion that is extreme and endures
- Fever or night sweats for no known explanation

Mouth changes

- A white or red fix on the tongue or in your mouth
- Bleeding and pain in the lip or mouth

Neurological issues

- Headaches
- Seizures
- Vision changes

- Hearing changes
- Drooping of the face

Skin changes

- A tissue shaded bump that drains or turns layered
- A new mole or an adjustment in a current mole
- A sore that doesn't recuperate
- Jaundice (yellowing of the skin and whites of the eyes)
- Growing or protuberances anyplace, for example, in the neck, underarm, stomach, and crotch
- putting on or weight reduction for no known explanation

Bladder changes

- Trouble urination
- Pain while urinating
- Blood in the urine

Draining or wounding, for no known explanation

Bowel changes

- Blood in the stools
- hinges in bowel propensities

Hack or dryness that doesn't leave

Eating problems

- Pain after eating (acid reflux or heartburn that doesn't go)
- Trouble gulping
- Belly torment
- Nausea and spewing
- Appetite changes
- Weakness that is extreme and keeps going
- Fever or night sweats for no known explanation

Neurological problems

- Headaches
- Seizures
- Vision changes
- Hearing changes
- Drooping of the face

5.**Diabetes mellitus**, ordinarily known as diabetes, is a metabolic infection that causes high glucose. The hormone insulin moves sugar from the blood into your cells to be put away or utilized for vitality. With diabetes, your body either doesn't make enough insulin or can't successfully use the insulin it makes.

Untreated high glucose from diabetes can harm your nerves, eyes, kidneys, and other organs.

There are a couple of various types of diabetes:

Type 1 diabetes: it is an immune system infection. The insusceptible framework assaults and annihilates cells in the pancreas, where insulin is made. It's hazy what causes this assault. Around 10 percent of individuals with diabetes have this type.

Type 2 diabetes: happens when your body gets impervious to insulin, and sugar develops in your blood.

Pre-diabetes happens when your glucose is higher than usual; however, it's not sufficiently high for a conclusion of type 2 diabetes.

Gestational diabetes: this result in high glucose during pregnancy—insulin-blocking hormones created by the placenta cause this type of diabetes.

The general symptoms of diabetes include:

- increased hunger
- increased thirst
- weight misfortune
- frequent pee
- blurry vision
- extreme exhaustion
- sores that don't recuperate

Obesity: This is an ailment where abundance muscle to fat ratio has gathered to the degree that it might negatively affect health.People are commonly viewed as fat when their weight file (BMI), an estimation acquired by isolating an individual's load by the square of the individual's stature, is more than 30 kg/m2; the range 25–30 kg/m2 is characterized as overweight. Some East Asian nations use lower esteems. Obesity improves the probability of different ailments and conditions, especially cardiovascular infections, type 2 diabetes, obstructive rest apnea, particular sorts of malignant growth, osteoarthritis, and sadness.

Obesity is a plague in the World. This condition puts individuals at a higher hazard for genuine illnesses. What's more, according to the Centers for Disease Control and Prevention (CDCP) "Factors, for example, age, sex, ethnicity, and bulk can impact the connection among BMI(Body Mass Index) and muscle versus fat. Additionally, BMI doesn't recognize overabundance fat, muscle, or bone mass, nor does it give any sign of the conveyance of fat among people."

Causes Of Obesity

Eating a much number of calories than you consume in day by day movement and exercise (on a long term premise) causes obesity. After some time, these additional calories include and cause you to put on weight.

Regular explicit reasons for obesity include:

- eating a less than stellar eating routine of nourishments high in fats and calories
- Having a stationary (dormant) way of life.
- You were not having enough sleeping, which can prompt hormonal changes that cause you to feel hungrier and want certain unhealthy nourishments.
- Genetics, which can influence how your body forms nourishment into vitality and how fat is put away.
- Growing more seasoned, which can prompt less bulk and a slower metabolic rate, making it simpler to put on weight.
- Pregnancy (weight picked up during pregnancy can be hard to lose and may inevitably prompt obesity).

Specific ailments may likewise prompt weight gain. These include:

- polycystic ovary disorder: a condition that causes an awkwardness of female regenerative hormones

- Prader-Willi disorder: an uncommon condition that an individual is brought into the world with which creates an unreasonable yearning
- Cushing disorder: a condition brought about by having an unnecessary measure of the hormone cortical in your framework
- hypothyroidism (underactive thyroid): a situation where the thyroid organ doesn't deliver enough of certain significant hormones
- osteoarthritis (and different conditions that cause torment that may prompt idleness).

Symptoms Of Obesity

Although increasing a couple of additional pounds may appear to be unimportant undoubtedly, weight addition can rapidly heighten to a genuine ailment.

Side effects of obesity can contrarily affect one's day by day life. For grown-ups, some symptom includes:

- Excess muscle versus fat amassing (especially around the midsection)
- Shortness of breath
- Sweating (more than expected)
- Snoring
- Trouble dozing
- Skin issues (from dampness collecting in the folds of skin)
- Inability to perform straightforward physical assignments (that one could without much of a stretch perform before weight gain)
- Fatigue (from gentle to extraordinary)
- Pain (generally in the back and joints)
- Psychological sway (negative confidence, sadness, disgrace, social seclusion)
- Eating issue
- Fatty tissue stores (might be perceptible in the bosom region)

- The appearance of stretch blemishes on the hips and back
- Acanthosis nigricans (dull smooth skin around the neck and different areas)
- Shortness of breath with physical action
- Sleep apnea
- Constipation
- GI reflux
- Poor confidence
- Early adolescence in young ladies/postponed pubescence in young men
- Orthopaedic issues, (for example, level feet or disjoined hips)

CHAPTER THREE

A COMPLETE GUIDE TO MINDFUL CHANGE AND RECOVERY FROM ANXIETY

Mindfulness implies keeping up minute-by-minute attention to our thoughts, feelings, substantial sensations, and general condition, through a delicate, supporting focal point.

Mindfulness additionally includes acknowledgement, implying that we focus on our thoughts and feelings without deciding between them—without accepting, for example, that there's a "right" or "wrong" approach to think or feel in a given minute. At the point when we practice mindfulness, our thoughts tune into what we're detecting right now instead of reiterating the past or envisioning what's to come.

BENEFITS OF MINDFULNESS

Mindfulness improves well-being.

Expanding your ability for mindfulness bolsters numerous perspectives that add to a fulfilled life. Being careful makes it simpler to relish the delights in life as they happen, causes you to become entirely occupied with exercises, and makes a more remarkable ability to manage unfavourable occasions. By concentrating on the present time and place, numerous individuals who practice mindfulness find that they are less inclined to become involved with stresses over the future or laments over the past, are less distracted with worries about progress and confidence, and are better ready to shape profound associations with others.

Mindfulness improves physical health.

On the off chance that more prominent well-being isn't sufficient of a motivating force, researchers have found that mindfulness strategies help improve physical health in various manners. Mindfulness can: help calm stress, treat coronary illness, lower circulatory strain, decrease incessant pain, improve rest, and mitigate gastrointestinal challenges.

Mindfulness improves mental health.

Lately, psychotherapists have gone to mindfulness contemplation as a significant component in the treatment of various issues, including melancholy, substance misuse, dietary issues, couples' contentions, anxiety issue, and over the top enthusiastic issue.

Analysts have discovered that IBMT (integrative body-mind preparing) starts necessary positive changes in the cerebrum that could help secure against mental sickness. The act of this system helps support productivity in a piece of the mind that assists individuals with managing conduct.

Mindfulness lightens some stress.

Since individuals are confronted with an expanding measure of weight nowadays because of the unpredictable idea of our general public, they are frequently tormented with a great deal of stress. This adds to a wide assortment of other health issues. Mindfulness can diminish stress by going about as a precaution measure, and assist individuals with overcoming troublesome occasions.

Mindfulness advances cognitive flexibility.

One examination recommends that not exclusively will mindfulness assist individuals with getting less receptive; it additionally may give individuals increasingly cognitive flexibility. Individuals who practice mindfulness give off an impression of being ready likewise to rehearse self-perception, which naturally separates the pathways made in the cerebrum from earlier learning, and permits data that is going on right now to be comprehended in another manner.

Mindfulness makes more happy relationships.

Analysts are as yet uncertain this works, yet rising cerebrum considers have demonstrated that individuals who take part in mindfulness all the time show both structural and functional changes in the mind areas that are connected to upgraded sympathy, empathy, and consideration.

Mindfulness diminishes anxiety.

Research has discovered that mindfulness is particularly useful in diminishing anxiety. Rehearsing mindfulness usually assists with revamping your cerebrum so you can pull together your consideration. Instead of following a negative and stressing thought down a way of every conceivable result, you can figure out how to perceive the truth about your feelings and let them go.

Mindfulness improvessleep.

The unwinding reaction that your body needs to mindfulness reflection is a remarkable inverse of the stress reaction. This unwinding reaction attempts to ease many stress-related health issues, for example, pain, despair, and hypertension. Rest issues are frequently attached to these afflictions.

Mindfulness gives pain relief.

Around 100 million Americans experience the ill effects of constant pain each day; however, 40% to 70% of these individuals are not accepting appropriate clinical treatment. Numerous examinations have demonstrated that mindfulness contemplation can diminish pain without utilizing endogenous narcotic frameworks that are typically allowed to decrease pain during cognitive-based procedures like mindfulness

CHAPTER ***FOUR***

ANXIETY

We, as a whole encounter anxiety; it is a natural human state and a crucial piece of our lives. Anxiety encourages us to distinguish and react to peril in 'battle or flight' mode. It can spur to us face up to managing troublesome difficulties. The 'perfect' measure of anxiety can assist us in performing a better and animate activity and innovativeness.

Be that as it may, there is another side to anxiety. Tireless anxiety causes genuine passionate distress and can prompt us getting unwell and, even under the least favourable conditions, creating anxiety issue, for example, alarm assaults, fears and fixation practices. Anxiety at this level can have a genuinely distressing and weakening effect on our lives and impact on our physical just as our mental health.

Anxiety is one of the most widely recognized mental health issues on the planet, and it is expanding. However, it stays under-detailed, under-analyzed and undertreated. A decent capacity to adapt to anxiety is critical to strength even with whatever life tosses at us. Notwithstanding, encountering it to an extreme or time after time implies we chance to turn out to be overpowered, incapable to discover balance in our lives or to unwind and recuperate. Our capacity to locate some inward harmony has never been progressively imperative to our well-being.

Everybody encounters anxiety. Be that as it may, when feelings of extreme dread and distress are overpowering and keep us from doing ordinary things.

Everybody has feelings of anxiety sooner or later in their life, regardless of whether it is tied in with getting ready for a prospective employee meeting, meeting an accomplice's family just because, or the possibility of parenthood. While we partner anxiety with modifications to our mental state, experienced as stress or trepidation maybe, and physical signs, for example, raised pulse and adrenaline, we additionally comprehend that it is probably going to influence us just briefly until the wellspring of our anxiety has passed or we have figured out how to adapt to it. Anxiety is in this way one of a scope of feelings that serves the positive capacity of making us aware of things we may need to stress over: possibly unsafe situations. All the more critically, these feelings help us to assess potential dangers and fittingly react to them, maybe by stimulating our reflexes or concentrating.

Anxiety is a word we use to depict feelings of disquiet, stress and dread. It consolidates both the feelings and the physical sensations we may encounter when we are stressed or apprehensive over something. Even though we, as a rule, think that it’s disagreeable, anxiety is identified with the 'battle or flight' reaction – our typical organic response to feeling compromised.

SYMPTOMS OF ANXIETY

Much the same as with any dysfunctional behaviour, individuals with anxiety issue experience indications in an unexpected way. Be that as it may, for the vast majority, anxiety changes how they work everyday. Individuals can encounter at least one of the accompanying side effects:

Excessive Worrying

One of the most widely recognized indications of an anxiety issue is excessive worrying.

The worrying related with anxiety issue is unbalanced to the occasions that trigger it and regularly happens in light of ordinary regular circumstances.

Worrying is dangerous and meddlesome, making it hard to think and achieve everyday undertakings.

Individuals younger than 65 are at the most noteworthy danger of summed up anxiety issue, particularly the single individuals, have a lower financial status and have numerous life stressors

Feeling Agitated

At the point when somebody is feeling on edge, some portion of their thoughtful sensory system goes into overdrive.

This commences a course of impacts all through the body, for example, a hustling beat, sweat-soaked palms, temperamental hands and dry mouth.

These side effects happen because your cerebrum trusts you have detected risk, and it is setting up your body to respond to the danger.

Your body shunts blood away from your stomach related framework and toward your muscles on the off chance that you have to run or battle. It likewise builds your pulse and elevates your faculties.

While these impacts would be useful on account of genuine risk, they can be debilitating if the fear is all in your mind.

Some examination even proposes that individuals with anxiety issue are not ready to diminish their excitement as fast as individuals without anxiety issue, which implies they may feel the impacts of anxiety for a more drawn out timeframe

Restlessness

Restlessness is another regular indication of anxiety, particularly in kids and youngsters.

At the point when somebody is encountering restlessness, they regularly depict it as feeling "tense" or having an "awkward inclination to move."

One investigation in 128 kids determined to have anxiety issue found that 74% revealed restlessness as one of their principle anxiety indications

Fatigue

Turning out to be effectively fatigued is another potential side effect of summed up an anxiety issue.

This side effect can be astonishing to a few, as anxiety is regularly connected with hyperactivity or excitement.

For a few, fatigue can follow an anxiety assault, while for other people, the fatigue can be chronic.

Difficulty InConcentrating

Numerous individuals with anxiety report experiencing issues concentrating.

A few examinations show that anxiety can intrude on working memory, a sort of memory answerable for holding momentary data. This may help clarify the emotional decline in execution individuals frequently experience during times of high anxiety.

Panic Attacks

One sort of anxiety issue called panic issue is related to repeating panic attacks.

Panic attacks produce an extreme, overpowering impression of fear that can be debilitating.

This extreme fear is regularly joined by quick heartbeat, sweating, shaking, and brevity of breath, chest snugness, queasiness and anxiety of biting the dust or losing control.

Panic attacks can occur in segregation; however, if they happen now and again and suddenly, they might be an indication of panic issue.

Maintaining a strategic distance from Social Situations

Individuals with social anxiety may show up incredibly timid and calm in gatherings or when meeting new individuals. While they may not seem upset outwardly, inside, they feel extraordinary fear and anxiety.

This detachedness can now and then cause individuals with social anxiety to seem vainglorious or standoffish; however, the turmoil is related to low confidence, high self-analysis and despondency.

You might be displaying indications of social anxiety issue if you get yourself:

- Feeling on edge or fearful about up and coming social circumstances
- Worried that you might be judged or examined by others
- Fearful of being humiliated or embarrassed before others
- Avoiding specific get-togethers in light of these fears

Irrational Fears

Unreasonable fears about specific things, for example, creepy crawlies, encased spaces or statures, could be an indication of fear.

Fear is characterized as excessive anxiety or worries about a particular item or circumstance. The feeling is serious enough that it meddles with your capacity to work typically.

TYPES OF ANXIETY DISORDER

Anxiety disorders have different indications or symptoms. This additionally implies each kind of anxiety has its treatment plan. The most widely recognized nervousness issue includes:

- **Panic Disorder**

  Panic disorder is an unexpected sentiment of terror;it strikes suddenly without warning.Physical side effects including chest pains, heart palpitations, unsteadiness, the brevity of breath and stomach upset.

- **Phobias**

  The vast majority with explicit fears have a few triggers. To abstain from freezing, somebody with understandable fears will strive to keep away from their triggers. Contingent upon the sort and number of triggers, this dread and the endeavour to control it can appear to assume control over an individual's life.

- **Generalized Anxiety Disorder (GAD)**

  GAD produces ceaseless, overstated agonizing over regular day to day existence. This can devour hours every day, making it difficult to focus or finish the routine day by day assignments. An individual with GAD may get depleted by stress and experience migraines, pressure or queasiness.

- **Social Anxiety Disorder**

  In contrast to modesty, this disorder causes extraordinary fear, regularly determined by unreasonable stresses over social embarrassment "saying something moronic," or "not recognizing what to state." Someone with a social anxiety disorder may pass on discussions, add to class conversations, or offer their thoughts, and may get secluded. The fit of anxiety side effects is a typical response.

- **Obsessive-Compulsive Disorder**

  Obsessive: Constant considerations, thoughts, motivations or pictures that are meddlesome and wrong and that cause checked anxiety or distress. People with fixations as a rule endeavour to disregard or smother such musings or driving forces or to balance them by different contemplations or activities (impulses).

  Compulsive: Repetitive practices, (for example, hand washing, requesting or checking) or mental acts, (for example, supplicating, tallying or rehashing words) that happen because of fixation or in a formal manner.

- **Post Traumatic Stress Disorder**

  This alludes to Flashbacks, steady startling musings and recollections, outrage or touchiness in light of a frightening involvement with which physical mischief happened or compromised, for example, (assault, child abuse, war or catastrophic event).

CAUSES OF ANXIETY DISORDER

Researchers accept that numerous components consolidate to cause anxiety disorders:

- **Genetics**

A few families will have a higher than reasonable quantities of individuals encountering anxiety issues, and studies bolster the proof that anxiety disorders run in families or hereditary. This can be a factor in somebody building up an anxiety disorder.

- **Stress**

A stressful or traumatic circumstance, for example, abuse, passing of a friend or family member, savagery or delayed sickness is regularly connected to the improvement of an anxiety disorder

IMPACTS OF ANXIETY ON THE BODY

Anxiety can create numerous uproars in your body as it gets ready for peril. These sensations are known as the "caution response", which happens when the body's regular Alarm System (the "battle flight-freeze" reaction) has been enacted.

Quick heartbeat and fast breathing – When your body is setting itself up for an activity, it ensures enough blood and oxygen is being coursed to your significant muscle gatherings and essential organs, permitting you to flee or ward off the threat.

Perspiring – Sweating cools the body. It likewise makes the skin increasingly tricky and hard for an assaulting creature or individual to grasp you.

Queasiness and stomach upset – When confronted with a threat, the body closes down frameworks/forms that are not required for endurance; that way, it can guide vitality to capacities that are basic for tolerance. Assimilation is one of the procedures that isn't needed on occasion of risk. Along these lines, anxiety may prompt sentiments of stomach upset, sickness, or lose bowels.

Feeling discombobulated or woozy – Because our blood and oxygen goes to significant muscle bunches when we are in harm's way; we inhale a lot quicker to push oxygen toward those muscles. Be that as it may, this reaction can cause hyperventilation (a lot of oxygen from breathing quickly to set up the body for activity), which can cause you to feel mixed up or unsteady. Likewise, since the vast majority of your blood and oxygen is setting off to your arms and legs (for "battle or flight"), there is a slight diminishing of blood to the cerebrum, which can likewise make you bleary-eyed. Try not to stress; however: the slight reduction in the blood stream to the mind isn't hazardous in any way.

Tight or agonizing chest – Your muscles worry as your body gets ready for the risk. So your chest may feel tight or difficult when you take in enormous breaths while those chest muscles are tense.

Deadness/numbness and shivering sensations – Hyperventilation (taking in excess of oxygen) can likewise create numbness and shivering uproars. The shivering sensations can also be identified with the way that the hairs on our bodies regularly stand up when confronted with risk to build our affectability to contact or development. At long last, fingers and toes may likewise feel numb/tingly as blood streams from places where it isn't required (like our fingers) and towards significant muscle bunches that are needed (like our arms).

The heaviness of legs - As the legs plan for activity (battle or flight), expanded muscle pressure, just as expanded blood stream to those muscles, can create the uproar of substantial legs.

Stifling or choking sensations – Increased muscle pressure around the neck or quick breathing dries out the throat, which may cause you to feel like you are gagging.

Hot and cold flashes – These sensations might be identified with perspiring and narrowing of veins in the upper skin layer. This narrowing likewise assists with decreasing blood loss if you are harmed.

Central nervous system

Long term anxiety and fits of stress can make your cerebrum discharge pressure hormones all the time. This can expand the recurrence of side effects, for example, cerebral pains, unsteadiness, and discouragement.

At the point when you felt on edge and focused on, your cerebrum floods your nervous system with hormones and synthetic compounds intended to assist you with reacting to a risk. Adrenaline and cortisol are two models.

While support for the periodic high-stress occasion, long term introduction to stretch hormones can be progressively hurtful to your physical wellbeing over the long term. For instance, long term introduction to cortical can add to weight gain.

Cardiovascular system

Anxiety disorders can cause fast pulse, palpitations, and chest torment or pains. You may likewise be at an expanded danger of hypertension and coronary illness. If you, as of now have coronary disease, anxiety disorders may raise the threat of coronary occasions.

Excretory and stomach related systems

Anxiety additionally influences your excretory and stomach related systems. You may have stomachaches, queasiness, looseness of the bowels, and other stomach related problems. Loss of craving can likewise happen.

There might be an association between anxiety disorders and the advancement of fractious inside disorder (IBS) after a gut disease. IBS can cause retching, the runs, or clogging.

The resistant or immune system

Anxiety can trigger your flight-or-battle pressure reaction and discharge a surge of synthetic concoctions and hormones, similar to adrenaline, into your system.

For the time being, this builds your heartbeat and breathing rate, so your mind can get more oxygen. This sets you up to react fittingly to an exceptional circumstance. Your safe system may even get a short lift. With infrequent pressure, your body comes back to typical working when the pressure passes.

On the off chance that you over and again felt on edge and focused or it keeps going quite a while, your body never gets the sign to come back to typical working. This can debilitate your immune system, leaving you increasingly helpless against viral diseases and incessant ailments. Likewise, your ordinary antibodies may not function too on the off chance that you have anxiety.

Respiratory system

Anxiety causes quick, shallow relaxing. If you have a constant obstructive aspiratory infection, you might be at an expanded danger of hospitalization from anxiety-related inconveniences. Anxiety can likewise exacerbate asthma signs.

other impacts

Anxiety disorder can cause different indications, including:

- Headaches
- muscle pressure
- insomnia
- depression
- social confinement

If you have PTSD (Post-traumatic stress disorder), you may encounter flashbacks, remembering a traumatic experience occasionally. Different side effects incorporate sleep deprivation, bad dreams, and trouble.

Yell it out

Conversing with a believed companion is one approach to adapt to anxiety. Be that as it may, there's something stunningly better than talking: shouting as loud as possible. As a child, you were presumably instructed not to yell and advised to utilize your "inside voice." But as a grown-up, you can make your principles. So in case you're managing repressed dissatisfactions and anxiety, let it out.

This doesn't mean bothering dread in others, so they feel like you. We're discussing a sound arrival of feelings in a controlled situation. The more you battle anxiety, the additionally overpowering it can turn into. Instead, hold onto fear as a piece of your life, and afterwards, let it go. Shout as loud as possible, punch a pad, step your feet, or pound your chest. Do whatever causes you to get it out! One Los Angeles-based yoga instructor even built up a class considered Tantrum Yoga that urges yogis to attempt these whimsical strategies as an approach to discharge feeling that "stalls out in our bodies and could transform into stress, illness, and so forth."

Get going

Exercise is most likely the exact opposite thing you need to do when your brain's in overdrive. You may stress over post-exercise irritation and being not able to walk or sit for the following two days. Or then again, your psyche may go to the direst outcome imaginable, and you dread overexerting yourself and having a coronary failure. Be that as it may,exercise is extraordinary compared to other common anti-anxiety arrangements.

Physical movement raises endorphins and serotonin levels to assist you with feeling better inwardly. Also, when you feel better within, your whole standpoint improves. What's more, because your cerebrum can't similarly concentrate on two things on the double, exercise can likewise take your brain off your issues. Focus on any event 30 minutes of physical movement three to five days every week. Try not to think you need to battle through an excruciating exercise. Any kind of development is acceptable, so put on your preferred jam and move around the house. Or then again get a tangle and break out into your preferred yoga presents.

Farewell to caffeine

Some espresso, chocolate, or a super cold Coke may assist you with feeling much improved. In any case, if caffeine is your go-to medication of decision, your anxiety could intensify.

Caffeine gives the sensory system a shock, which supports vitality levels. Be that as it may, when under tension, this anxious vitality can instigate an anxiety assault. Presently, surrendering your most loved stimulated refreshment may raise your pulse and prompt anxiety as you read this, yet you don't need to plug without any weaning period or surrender caffeine. It's everything about control.

Instead of four cups of espresso daily, downsize to a couple of ordinary estimated cups a day — typical as in 8 ounces, not 16 or 32 ounces. Give it a trial and perceive how you feel. As you wean yourself, gradually bring different drinks into your eating regimen, for example, decaffeinated natural tea, which can quiet your brain and nerves.

Give yourself a sleeping time

With your bustling calendar, there's no time for rest, correct? A few compulsive workers gloat about just requiring three or four hours of rest a night, as though to state, "I'm more decided and submitted than every other person." But regardless of what you may let yourself know, you're not a robot. People need rest to work appropriately, so except if you radiated in from some close by planet, this additionally concerns you.

Regardless of whether you manage a sleeping disorder, deliberately limit your measure of rest, or you're a self-purported night owl, constant lack of sleep makes you helpless to anxiety. Do yourself (and everybody around you) some favour and get eight to nine hours of rest each night. Build up a sleep time routine to peruse a book or accomplish something unwinding before bed. The better set you up are to get a decent night's rest, the better nature of rest you'll have, which prompts a superior morning too.

Feel “OK”saying ” NO“

Your plate is just so enormous, and on the off chance that you overpower yourself with every other person's very own issues, your anxiety will likewise decline. We've all heard the saying, "There's more joy in giving than accepting." But no place right now it states you ought to kick back and let others encroach on your time.

Regardless of whether you're driving somebody around on tasks, getting their children from school, or listening attentively about their issues, you'll have little solidarity to think about your problems on the off chance that you burn through practically the entirety of your effort thinking about others. This doesn't mean you ought never to support anybody, however, know your confinements, and don't be hesitant to state "no" when you have to.

Try not to skip dinners

If anxiety causes queasiness, the idea of eating nourishment is as engaging as eating earth. Be that as it may, skipping suppers can aggravate anxiety. Your glucose drops when you don't eat, which causes the arrival of a stress hormone called cortisol. Cortisol can assist you with performing better under tension, yet it can likewise aggravate you feel in case you're as of now inclined to anxiety.

The way that you have to eat doesn't legitimize stuffing only anything in your mouth, so this isn't a reason to revel in sugar and shoddy nourishment. Sugar doesn't cause anxiety, yet a sugar surge can cause physical signs of anxiety, for example, apprehension and shaking. Also, on the off chance that you start to fixate on a response to sugar, you could have an out-all fit of anxiety.

Join increasingly lean proteins, natural products, vegetables, and solid fats into your eating regimen. Eat five to six little suppers for the day, and maintain a strategic distance from or limit your admission of sugar and refined starches.

Give yourself an exit strategy

Here and there, anxiety is because of feeling wild. You can't generally be in the driver seat of your life; however, you can find a way to distinguish your triggers and adapt to conditions that cause anxiety.

Does the idea of going into a social circumstance or meeting new individuals make you need to hop off an extension? As everybody at a gathering takes part in energizing discussions, perhaps you see yourself holding up the divider and checking during the time until you're put out of your wretchedness. You drove with companions and can't leave, so you spend the whole evening resembling the punchbowl orderly. It's this dread makes you decrease solicitations and rest as the weekends progressed.

Yet, imagine a scenario where you had a leave system set up before going out. For instance, rather than carpooling with your hardcore partier companions, you could drive yourself. Along these lines, you can leave if your anxiety begins to assemble and you can't deal with one more moment of clumsy associations. The more in charge you feel, the less anxiety you'll have.

CHAPTER FIVE

PANIC ATTACKS

Panic attacks are unexpected times of serious dread that may incorporate palpitations, sweating, shaking, the brevity of breath, numbness, or an inclination that something terrible will occur. The most extreme level of indications happens in no time. Commonly they keep going for around 30 minutes; however, the term can change from seconds to hours. There might be a dread of losing control or chest pain. Panic attacks themselves are not ordinarily risky genuinely.

Panic attacks can happen because of various disorders, including panic disorder, social anxiety disorder, post-traumatic stress disorder, tranquillize use disorder, wretchedness, and clinical problems. They can either be activated or happen suddenly. Smoking, caffeine, and mental stress increment the danger of having a panic attack. Before analysis, conditions that produce comparative side effects ought to be precluded, for example, hyperthyroidism, hyperparathyroidism, coronary illness, and lung illness.

REASONS FOR PANIC ATTACKS

Despondency

Despondency is named a temperament disorder. It might be depicted as sentiments of bitterness, misfortune, or outrage that meddle with an individual's ordinary exercises.

Alcohol abuse

Alcohol abuse includes a range of unfortunate alcohol drinking practices, going from hitting the bottle hard to alcohol reliance, in extreme cases bringing about medical issues for people and enormous scope social issues.

Cigarette smoking

Cigarette smoking is the act of smoking tobacco and breathing in tobacco smoke (comprising of the molecule and vaporous stages). A more extensive definition may incorporate just taking tobacco smoke into the mouth, and afterwards discharging it, as is finished by some with tobacco funnels and stogies.

Suicide hazard

Suicide is the demonstration of ending one's own life. As indicated by the American Foundation for Suicide Prevention, suicide is the tenth driving reason for death in the United States, ending the lives of around 47,000 Americans every year.

Self-destructive conduct alludes to discussing or taking activities identified with taking one's own life. Self-destructive musings and practices ought to be viewed as a mental crisis.

Hereditary qualities

A few families will have a higher than reasonable quantities of individuals encountering panic issues, and studies bolster the proof that panic disorders run in families. This can be a factor in somebody building up an anxiety disorder.

SIDE EFFECTS OF PANIC ATTACKS

Panic attacks commonly start of nowhere, all of a sudden. They can strike whenever – when you're driving a vehicle, at the shopping centre, sound snoozing or in a conference. You may have periodic panic attacks, or they may happen now and again.

Panic attacks have numerous varieties, yet signs as a rule top in no time. You may feel exhausted and exhausted after a panic attack dies down.

Panic attacks ordinarily incorporate a portion of these signs or indications:

- Sense of approaching fate (IMPENDING DOOM) or threat
- Fear of loss of control or death
- The rapid, beating pulse
- Sweating
- Trembling or shaking
- Shortness of breath or snugness in your throat
- Chills
- Hot flashes
- Nausea
- Abdominal squeezing
- Chest pain
- Headache
- Dizziness, tipsiness or faintness

- Numbness or shivering sensation
- Feeling of falsity or separation.

IMPACT OF PANIC ATTACKS

People, who experience the ill effects of panic disorder, or panic attacks, might be at a lot higher danger of coronary episode and coronary illness sometime down the road. ... During these attacks, individuals may likewise encounter physical signs, including perspiring, breathing issues, tipsiness, dashing heart, hot or cold chills, chest torment and stomach torment.

Long term anxiety and panic attacks can make your cerebrum discharge stress hormones all the time. This can expand the recurrence of side effects, for example, cerebral pains, discombobulating, and grief.

Panic attacks during pregnancy can be a reason for concern since they can affect the hatchling. Bloodstream to the hatchling is diminished when their moms are encountering high anxiety, which can prompt low birth weight and early work.

Individuals with panic disorder may have cerebrums that are particularly delicate in reacting to fear. Individuals with this disorder regularly additionally have significant sadness.

Panic attacks can influence the mother-youngster relationship and a mother's capacity to adapt in the postpartum period.

SOLUTION TO PANIC ATTACKS

As signs top during a panic attack, it can feel like the experience will never end. While you may believe there's nothing you can do aside from enduring it, there are a few procedures you can practice to lessen the seriousness of your signs and divert your psyche.

Perceive that you have a panic attack

By perceiving that you're having a panic attack rather than a coronary episode, you can advise yourself this is brief, it will pass, and that you're OK.

Remove the dread that you might be kicking the bucket or that approaching fate is approaching, the two signs of panic attacks. This can permit you to concentrate on different systems to decrease your side effects.

Have a Plan in Place

Regardless of what your arrangement is, having one set up is the most significant thing. You can think about your arrangement as your go-to set of directions for yourself when you feel a panic attack going ahead. One mechanism may be to remove yourself from your present condition, plunk down, and consider a companion or relative that can help occupy you from your indications and help you to quiet down. At that point, you can join the accompanying systems.

Practice Deep Breathing

The brevity of breath is a typical indication of panic attacks that can cause you to feel berserk and wild. Recognize that your shortness of breath is a sign of a panic attack, and this is just transitory. At that point start by taking a full breath in for a sum of four seconds, hold for a second, and discharge it for an amount of four seconds. Continue rehashing this example until your breathing gets controlled and consistent. Concentrating on the tally of four not exclusively will keep you from hyperventilating; however, it can likewise assist with leaving different side effects speechless.

Practice mindfulness

Mindfulness can help ground you in the truth of what's around you. Since panic attacks can cause a sentiment of separation or partition from the real world, this can battle your panic attack as its drawing closer or occur.

Concentrate on the physical sensations you know about, such as delving your feet into the ground or feeling the surface of your pants on your hands. These particular sensations ground you immovably actually and give you something goal to concentrate on.

Use Muscle Relaxation Techniques

Amidst a panic attack, it's unavoidable that you'll feel like you've lost control of your body, yet muscle unwinding methods permit you to recover a portion of that control. Dynamic muscle unwinding is a straightforward, however powerful strategy for panic and anxiety disorders. Start by gripping your clench hand and holding this grasp until the tally of 10. When you find a workable pace, the hold and let your hand unwind totally. Next, attempt a similar strategy in your feet, and afterwards, bit by bit stir your way up your body grasping and loosening up each muscle gathering: legs, excesses, stomach area, back, hands, arms, shoulders, neck, and face.

Participate in light exercise

Endorphins keep the blood siphoning in precisely the immediately. It can help flood our body with endorphins, which can improve our temperament. Since you're stressed, pick a light exercise that is delicate on the body, such as strolling or swimming. The particular case to this is in case you're hyperventilating or attempting to relax. Do what you can to slow down first.

Rehash or repeat a Mantra

You may feel somewhat clumsy doing this from the outset however rehashing an empowering, positive mantra to yourself during a panic attack can fill in as a way of dealing with stress. Take stab at repeating something as straightforward as "This is transitory. I will be alright," or "I'm not going to kick the bucket. I need to relax."

Discover an Object and Focus on It

Pick an item that you can see someplace before you and note all that you notice about that object—from its shading and size to any examples it might have, where you may have seen others like it, or what something different to the article would resemble. You can do this in your mind or talk your observational resoundingly to yourself or a companion.

Close your eyes

Some panic attacks originate from triggers that overpower you. In case you're in a quick-paced condition with a lot of improvements, this can take care of your panic attack.

To diminish the improvements, close your eyes during your panic attack. This can shut out any additional upgrades and make it simpler to concentrate on your relaxing.

Picture your cheerful spot

What's the most loosening up place on the planet that you can consider? A bright seashore with delicately moving waves? Or A lodge in the mountains?

Imagine yourself there, and attempt to concentrate on the subtleties however much as could reasonably be expected. Envision delving your toes into the warm sand, or smelling the sharp fragrance of pine trees. This spot ought to hush up, quiet, and to unwind.

Maintain a strategic distance from 'self sedating or medication.'

Attempt to maintain a strategic distance from "self sedating". Alcohol won't help sentiments of panic, and in the long term, will aggravate them. Tranquillizers here and there have an extremely transient use, yet they are not valuable in the more extended time and it is anything but difficult to get dependent. Know that a few drugs for anxiety can be addictive - consistently get clinical exhortation about any meds.

Chapter SIX

ANGER

The emotion of anger is not always a negative feeling to experience. Being angry in some ways can be a positive outlet and something that should not be ignored.

In any case, having rage inside that outcomes in destructive inclinations towards yourself or others, and from which the source is a painful experience, isn't healthy in any way. This sort of anger ought to be managed before it grows into progressively negative encountersanger/rage is at last your companion and close partner. In any case, until you can acknowledge this feeling like a piece of your being, you will, in general, be at war with the feeling of anger just as yourself. You should initially comprehend that anger is a defensive feeling and afterwards consider the manners by which anger can be valuable and favourable to you. Since anger or fierceness springs quickly from torment and dread, and later eventually love, you should be cautious that this anger isn't disengaged from other essential feelings. This is the point at which it gets dangerous. When you exceed that limit of thinking about your sentiments or the sentiments of someone else, your anger can ingrain torment, either passionate or physical. Then again, on the off chance that you can interface love for each irate inclination you get, anger will in general break down and love and sense win.

Anger is one of the most fundamental human feelings. It is a physical and mental reaction to a danger or to hurt done before. Anger takes a wide range of structures from aggravation to blinding fierceness or disdain that rots over numerous years. Anytime, a blend of physical, mental and social components interface to cause us to feel a specific way. It's distinctive for every one of us. Our sentiments are impacted by our passionate make-up, how we see the world, what occurs around us and our conditions. Like different feelings, anger once in a while demonstrations alone.

SORTS OF ANGER

Uninvolved or passive Anger

Individuals encountering uninvolved anger may not understand they are irate. At the point when you experience aloof anger, your feelings might be shown as mockery, aloofness or unpleasantness. You may take an interest in reckless practices, for example, playing hooky or work, distancing loved ones, or performing inadequately in expert or social circumstances. To untouchables, it will seem as though you are purposefully subverting yourself, even though you may not understand it or have the option to clear your activities.

Since inactive anger might be quelled, it very well may be difficult to perceive; advising can assist you with recognizing the feelings behind your activities, exposing the object of your anger so you can manage it.

Forceful or aggressive Anger

People who experience forceful anger are typically mindful of their feelings, even though they don't generally comprehend the genuine underlying foundations of their rage. Sometimes, they divert violent anger upheavals to substitutes since it is too hard to even think about dealing with real issues. Forceful anger regularly shows as unstable or retaliatory anger and can bring about physical harms to property and others. Figuring out how to perceive triggers and oversee anger indications is fundamental to managing this type of anger.

Assertive Anger

The sound method to manage anger is by being controlled and confident, listening and talking, and open to help in managing the situation. This Assertive anger can assist associations with growing. It implies thinking before you talk, being positive about how you state it, yet open and adaptable to the 'opposite side.' It implies showing restraint, not raising your voice, imparting how you are feeling inwardly, and truly attempting to comprehend what others are feeling. At the point when you manage anger assertively, you show that you are fully grown and care about your connections and yourself.

HOW ANGER WORKS

As we go about our lives, we're continually weighing up circumstances and choosing our opinion of them: positive or negative, protected or perilous and so forth how we decipher a circumstance impacts how we feel about it. If we think a circumstance signifies 'you are in danger', we feel apprehensive. On the off chance that it means 'you have been wronged', we feel furious. Also, these emotions decide how we respond to the circumstance. We make an interpretation of implications into sentiments quick. With anger, that speed in some cases implies that we respond in a way we later regret. From the minute we are conceived, we are watching occasions, giving them implications and making a relationship between them. From our experience, we figure out how to evaluate every circumstance.

THE NATURE OF ANGER

Anger is an enthusiastic express that shifts in power from mellow bothering to extreme fierceness and wrath. Like different feelings, it is joined by physiological and natural changes. At the point when you blow up, your pulse and circulatory strain go up, as do the degrees of your vitality hormones, adrenaline, and nor-adrenaline. Anger can be brought about by both outer and inside occasions. You could resent a particular individual (colleague or manager at your working environment) or occasion (car influx, dropped flight), or your anger could be brought about by stressing or agonizing over your issues. Recollections of traumatic or chafing occasions can likewise trigger irate sentiments.

HOW OUR BODIES RESPOND TO ANGER

Vast numbers of our feelings are connected to a specific physical reaction. Anger prepares the psyche and body for activity. It stirs the sensory system, expanding the pulse, circulatory strain, bloodstream to muscles, glucose level and perspiring. It additionally hones the faculties and expands the creation of adrenalin, a hormone delivered on occasion of stress. Simultaneously as these physical changes, anger is thought to influence how we feel or believe. At the point when we are first confronted with danger, anger encourages us to rapidly interpret complex data into straightforward terms: 'right' or 'wrong' for example. This can be helpful in a crisis as we don't burn through significant time, weighing up data that doesn't right away influence our security or prosperity. In any case, it can imply that we demonstration before we've thought about what else is significant and settled on a balanced choice about how to act. It might be that we have to set aside more effort to take a gander at the circumstance and manage it unexpectedly. At the point when anger hinders objective reasoning, we may offer a path to the inclination to act forcefully, moved by the impulse to endure or shield somebody from a risk.

REASONS WHY PEOPLE GET ANGRY

Sentiments of anger emerge because of how we decipher and respond to specific circumstances. Everybody has their triggers for what drives them mad, yet some basic ones remember circumstances for which we feel.

Individuals can unexpectedly decipher circumstances, so a situation that drives you to feel extremely crazy may not force another person feel mad by any means (for instance, different responses could incorporate inconvenience, hurt or diversion). Be that as it may, because we can unexpectedly decipher things, it doesn't imply that you're interpreting things 'wrong' on the off chance that you blow up.

How you decipher and respond to a circumstance can rely upon bunches of variables in your life, including:

- adolescence and upbringing
- past encounters
- current conditions
- Hurt
- Threatened
- Not in control

Adolescence/Upbringing: Almost positively, how you were raised, and your social foundation, will impact how you feel about communicating anger. Numerous individuals are, as youngsters, given messages about anger that may make it harder to oversee as a grown-up.

You may have been raised to accept that it is in every case alright to showcase your anger, maybe forcefully or brutally, and not instructed how to comprehend and oversee it. This could mean you have furious upheavals whenever you don't care for how somebody is carrying on, or you are in a circumstance you don't care for.

Be that as it may, on the off chance that you had seen your folks' or other grown-ups' anger when it was crazy, you may have considered it to be something ruinous and alarming.

Or on the other hand, you may have been raised to accept that you ought not to whine yet oughtrather endure things, and may have been rebuffed for communicating anger as a youngster.

Encounters like these can imply that you stifle your anger and it turns into a long term issue, where you respond improperly to new circumstances you are not happy with.

Past Encounters: If you've encountered specific circumstances in the past that drove you to feel mad, for example, abuse, injury or harassing (either as a kid or all the more as of late as a grown-up), and you couldn't securely communicate your anger at that point, you may, in any case, be adapting to those irate sentiments now. This may imply that you currently discover certain circumstances especially testing, and bound to drive you crazy.

At times your present sentiment of anger may not exclusively be about the current circumstance yet may likewise be identified with a past encounter, which can imply that the anger you are feeling in the present is at a level that mirrors your past circumstance.

Getting mindful of this can assist us with finding methods for reacting to circumstances in the present in a more secure and less distressed manner.

Current conditions: In case you're managing a ton of different issues in your life at this moment, you may wind up feeling furious more effectively than expected, or blowing up at random things.

If there's specific that is driving you to feel mad; however, you don't feel ready to communicate your anger legitimately or resolve it, at that point you may discover you express that anger at different occasions.

Anger can likewise be a piece of pain. On the off chance that you've lost somebody essential to you, it very well may be colossally hard to adapt to all the clashing things you may be feeling.

Hurt: Individuals are regularly either be mindful and adoring towards us or mean and harmful.

Threatened:We feel this when there's a risk to our self-character, for example, the chance of being viewed as off-base, terrible, second rate or frail.

Anger influences various pieces of your body, including your heart, cerebrum, and muscles. An examination found that anger likewise causes an expansion in testosterone levels and lessening in cortical levels.

Not in Control: Feeling in charge is a characteristic human want and one that is significantly increasingly critical to specific individuals.

Depression

There is, by all accounts, a misconception that depression is continuously crying and not getting up." However, expanded crabbiness is a typical cause of anger.

Anxiety

People with high anxiety frequently feel very nearly overpowering because they need to make a substantial effort to deal with their inward enthusiastic state." So when a difficult circumstance emerges, you may be pushed to the limit, which shows as anger or a short circuit.

Alcohol Abuse

Alcohol abuse, or alcoholism, alludes to expending a lot of alcohol immediately or usually.

Research shows that drinking alcohol expands hostility.

Alcohol weakens your capacity to think unmistakably and settle on balanced choices. It influences your motivation control and can make it harder for you to control your feelings.

Bipolar Disorder

Bipolar disorder is a mental disorder that causes emotional moves in your disposition.

This extreme state of mind movements can extend from insanity to depression, in spite of the fact that not every person with bipolar disorder will encounter depression. In any case, many individuals with bipolar disorder may encounter times of anger, fractiousness, and wrath.

Intermittent Explosive Disorder

An individual with the intermittent explosive disorder (IED) has rehashed scenes of forceful, rash, or vicious conduct. They may go overboard to circumstances with irate upheavals that are out of extent to the circumstance.

Grief

Grief is one of the reasons for anger. Pain can emerge out of the death of a friend or family member, a separation or divorce from your love ones, or from losing a job. The anger might be aimed at the individual who passed on, any other person engaged with the occasion, or lifeless things.

HOW ANGER LEAD TO VIOLENCE

Anger can give an enormous flood of vitality that causes you to respond in manners that you regularly would not. At the point when it gains out of power, it transforms into a rage that can have negative ramifications for you and people around you.

If you are encountering incredible feelings, this can likewise trigger savage emotions. These feelings can be exacerbated, and are bound to prompt savagery, on the off chance that you drink excessively or abuse drugs.

The outcomes of letting your anger transform into brutality make it much increasingly significant for you to keep up control and find support with dealing with your emotions.

IMPACTS OF ANGER

Ceaseless anger that constantly erupts or spirals crazy can have negative ramifications for you're:

It debilitates your immune system.

In case you're distraught constantly, you could wind up feeling debilitated all the more frequently. In one examination, Harvard University researchers found that in reliable individuals, just reviewing a furious encounter from their past caused a six-hour dunk in levels of the counteracting agent immunoglobulin A, the cells' first line of resistance against disease.

Physical-wellbeing

Continually working at significant levels of stress and anger makes you increasingly defenceless to coronary illness, diabetes, a debilitated safe framework, a sleeping disorder, and hypertension.

Psychological wellness

Chronic anger expends large measures of mental vitality, and mists your reasoning, making it harder to focus or appreciate life. It can likewise prompt stress, gloom, and other psychological wellness issues,

Vocation or career

Constructive analysis, innovative contrasts, and heated discussion can be healthy. However, lashing out estranges your associates, supervisors, or customers and dissolves their respect,

Relationships

Anger can cause enduring scars in your loved ones most and hinder fellowships and work connections. Hazardous anger makes it difficult for others to confide in you, talk honestly, or feel good—and is particularly harming to youngsters.

If you have a hot temper, you may feel like it's out of your hands and there's little you can do to tame the brute. In any case, you have more authority over your anger than you might suspect. With understanding about the good explanations behind your anger and these anger the board instruments, you can figure out how to communicate your feelings without harming others and shield your temper from commandeering your life.

SYMPTOMS OF ANGER

Anger also causes some physical and emotional symptoms. While it's entirely expected to encounter these symptoms every so often, an individual with anger issues will, in general, experience them all the more frequently and to an increasingly extreme degree.

Interrupting

Angry individuals will, in general, be impatient individuals. Frequently they have inconvenient waiting for others to finish what they are saying. And in any event, when they can let the other people talk, they may not be listening in – but just pretending to be.

Being a Complainer

Individuals who invest a ton of energy complaining about the transgressions and shortcomings of other individuals may have an anger "issue.

Irritability

it is an unnecessary reaction to stimuli. The term is utilized for both the physiological response to stimuli and for the obsessive, strange or exorbitant affectability to stimuli; It is generally used to allude to anger or disappointment. Irritability might be exhibited in conduct reactions to both physiological and conduct stimuli, including natural, situational, sociological, and passionate stimuli.

Holding a Grudge

Relationships can endure when somebody has inconvenient forgiving somebody who has wronged him/her in the past. And individuals with anger issues frequently have inconvenience doing only that.

Instead, they continue to re-experience the frustration, hatred and pain each time they recall an inappropriate - whether saw or real.

Muscle strain

Is the extending or tearing of muscle fibres? Most muscle strains occur for one of two reasons: either the muscle has been extended past its breaking points, or it has been compelled to contract too unequivocally. In gentle cases, just a couple of muscle fibres are extended or torn, and the muscle stays flawless and solid. In severe cases, be that as it may, the strained muscle might be torn and unfit to work appropriately.

Red In The Face

Getting angry get the facial expression- and that goes for emotional "heat" as well as hot temperatures as measured on a thermometer. Anger can also cause labour breathing, fidgeting, and in any event, pacing back and forward.

Anger impacts the body as well as the mind. In fact, various investigations have indicated that angry individuals are bound to have hypertension and to endure a stroke or heart attack.

Shouting

This is the act of talking with frustration and to speak with a loud voice, frequently as boisterous as would be prudent, normally when you need to make yourself understood in loud circumstances, or when the individual you are conversing with is far away or can't hear well indeed and its somehow happen when you are angry, and it can lead to conflicts

Being Overly Sensitive

Angry individuals are speedy to take offence. Remarks that others may laugh off can get under the skin of somebody who has an angry demeanour. A few people with an anger "issue" are hyper-vigilant, always waiting for others to mess up.

Being Cold-Hearted

Angry individuals tend not to be extremely compassionate or empathetic. Some take pleasure in the adversity of others – an incident known as schadenfreude. And some are speedy to sentence and delayed to praise.

EFFECTS OF ANGER

Physical effects of anger

Anger triggers the body's 'battle or flight' reaction. Different feelings that trigger this reaction incorporate dread, energy, and uneasiness. The adrenal organs flood the body with pressure hormones, for example, adrenaline and cortical. The cerebrum shunts blood away from the gut and towards the muscles in anticipation of physical effort. Pulse, circulatory strain, and breath increment, the internal heat level ascents, and the skin sweats. The psyche is honed and centred.

Health problems with anger

The consistent surge of pressure synthetics and related metabolic changes that go with continuous unmanaged anger can, in the long run, cause mischief to various frameworks of the body.

A portion of the short and long haul health problems that have been connected to unmanaged anger include:

- Headache
- Digestion problems, for example, stomach torment
- Insomnia
- Increased nervousness
- Depression
- High circulatory strain

- Skin problems, for example, dermatitis
- Heart assault
- Stroke

HOW TO OVERCOME ANGER

Ready to get your anger levelled out? Start by considering these anger management tips.

Think before speaking

In the moment of being angry, it's easy to say something you'll later regret. Take a few seconds to gather your considerations or thoughts before saying anything — and allow others involved in the situation to do likewise.

Once calmed, express your anger

Immediately you're thinking clearly, express your frustration in an assertive but non-confrontational way. Mention your concerns and needs clearly and directly, without hurting others or trying to control them.

Take a breather

Your breathing may become shallower and accelerates as you become angry. You can reverse that trend (and your anger) by taking moderate, exhaling out of your mouth and full breaths from your nose for several moments.

Get some exercise

Physical activity can help reduce the stress that can cause you to lose control. If you feel your anger escalating, take a brisk walk or run, or invest some energy doing other enjoyable physical activities.

By relaxing your muscle

Dynamic muscle relaxation calls on you to tense and gradually relax various muscle bunches in your body, each in turn. As you tense and release, take moderate, deliberate breaths.

Take some time-out

Time-outs are not just for kids or children. Give yourself short breaks during times of the day that tend to be stressful. A couple of seconds of quiet time might help you feel better prepared to handle what's ahead without getting irritated or angry.

Identify some possible or potential solutions

Instead of focusing on what makes you angry or vex, chip away at resolving the issue at hand. Does your child's chaotic room drive you crazy? Close the entryway. Is your partner late for dinner consistently? Calendar meals later in the evening — or agree to eat on your own a couple of times seven days. Remind yourself that anger cannot fix anything and might just make it more regrettable.

Repeat some mantra

Find a phrase or word that helps you refocus and calm down. Say that word again and again to yourself when you're angry.

"Relax,""You'll be OK," and "Take it easy, are all genuine examples.

Intellectually escape

Walk into a quiet room, close your eyes, and practice visualizing yourself in a relaxing scene. Concentrate on details in the imaginary scene: How large are the mountains? How are the birds chirping sound like? This practice can help you find calm amidst anger.

Limit your word

At the point when you're steamed, you might be enticed to let the furious words fly, but you'll be more likely to do harm than great. Pretend your lips are stuck shut, just like you did as a kid or child. Some moments without speaking will give you time to collect your thoughts.

Stick with 'I' statements

To avoid placing blame or criticizing — which might just increase tension — use "I" statements to describe the issue. Be specific and respectful. For example, say, "I'm vexed that you left the table without offering to help with the dishes" rather than "You never do any housework."

Don't hold a grudge

Forgiveness is an incredible asset. If you allow negative feelings and anger to swarm out positive feelings, you might find yourself swallowed up by your feelings or bitterness of injustice. But if you are able to forgive someone who angered you, you might both learn from the situation and strengthen your relationship.

Use humour to release tension

Lightening up can help to diffuse tension. Humour helps to face what's making you angry and, possibly, any unrealistic expectations you have for how things ought to go. Avoid sarcasm, though it can hurt feelings and make things more regrettable.

Practice relaxation skills

At the point when your emotion flares, put relaxation skills to work. Practice profound breathing exercises, imagine a relaxing scene, or repeat a calming word or phrase, for example, "Take it easy." You might write in a journal, listen to music, or do a couple of yoga presents – whatever it takes to encourage relaxation.

Know when to seek help

Learning how to control our emotions is a challenge for everybody at times. Seek advice for anger issues. If your passion appears to be out of control, it can lead you to do things you regret or hurts those around you.

Forgiveness

Forgiveness is always important; if an individual has apologized or begged for making you angry, or if you realize that the situation "isn't worth it," be available to forgive. And willing to be forgiven and forgive yourself! It will help you to calm down and will help your relationships with others to flourish.

Practice empathy

Try to walk in the other individual's shoes and see the situation from their perspective or experience. When you tell the story or relive the events as they saw it, you may gain another understanding and become less angry.

Express your anger

It's OK to say what you feel, as long as you can handle it in the right way. Ask a trusted friend to help you to be accountable and calm to the response. Outbursts take care of no issues, but mature dialogue can help reduce your stress and ease your anger. It may also prevent the future.

Laugh

Nothing overturns a bad state of mind like a decent one. Diffuse your anger by looking for ways to smile, whether that's playing with your kids, watching stand-up, or scrolling images.

Practice gratitude

Take a moment to concentrate on what's right when everything feels wrong. Realizing what number of beneficial things you have in your life can help you neutralize anger and turn around the situation.

Talking therapy and counselling

This involves talking about your issues with a trained professional (for example, a guide or psychotherapist) who can help you explore the causes of your anger and ways to manage it. This can help you work through your feelings and improve your responses to situations that make you angry.

www.ingramcontent.com/pod-product-compliance
Lightning Source LLC
Chambersburg PA
CBHW070438271225
37375CB00015B/761
9781803474014